Green

Smoothies

For Seniors

Copyright © 2016 Argon Media, LLC

Disclaimer

All the material contained in this book is provided for educational and informational purposes only. No responsibility can be taken for any results or outcomes resulting from the use of this material.

While every attempt has been made to provide information that is both accurate and effective, the author does not assume any responsibility for the accuracy or use/misuse of this information.

You are encouraged to print this book for easy reading.

Use this information at your own risk.

Contents

Preface

If you are a senior looking to improve your health it can be a daunting task. Where do you start? With your doctor is the best first step. But even before that, just beginning to take note of what you eat every day will pay off quicker than anything else.

One of the best ways to get a nutritious lift is to start drinking smoothies for seniors. This little secret is responsible for adding tons of nutrient dense foods into your diet in a very digestible way - raw.

Raw fruits, vegetables, seeds and nuts have proven to be the best building blocks for supplying your body with daily nutrients not found anywhere else that is ultra-convenient.

According to research by the Harvard School of Public Health they explain: "it's hard to argue with the health benefits...of a diet rich in vegetables and fruits: Lower blood pressure; reduced risk of heart disease; stroke and probably some cancers; lower risk of eye and digestive problems; and a mellowing effect on blood sugar that can help keep appetite in check."

Inside of this manual, Green Smoothies for Seniors, you will get an up close and personal look at what to do to make adding smoothies to your daily life as easy as possible.

This guide focuses on the quickest and easiest ways to get this new habit up and working in your life.

Before we begin, it is important to note that you are much older now than you were years ago in your youth. You have years of accumulated habits that can be changed over time, but it is important to be patient with yourself.

If you try one fruit or vege and not find it to your liking, just substitute an alternative fruit or vegetable. You will want to keep an open mind. And remember according to WebMD, "Experts say a diet rich in fruits and vegetables can help you ward off infections like colds and flu." That means you'll be avoiding the problem most Americans have of not getting enough fruits and vegetables every day.

Introduction

"Even if you're on the right track, you'll get run over if you just sit there."

- Mark Twain

There is an old proverb that says, "Health is a crown on a well man's head that no one sees but a sick man."

This is very true. We live in a very hectic world today where everyone is focused on building a successful career and raising a happy family. They often place their health on the backburner, thinking that they can exercise and eat right later on.

They procrastinate exercise waiting till they're successful or have time to spare. They opt for quick, unhealthy meals because they have no time to prepare well-balanced meals.

They fail to realize that if you don't make time for exercise, you must make time for illness. They forget that whatever they eat and drink is either fighting disease or feeding it.

Today, more than ever, one needs to focus on his or her health and well-being. It is crucial. Our lives are filled with deadlines, meetings, work demands and stress. The food we eat is high in calories but low in nutrients.

High carbohydrate meals, oily and fatty foods, processed foods, junk food, etc. wreak havoc on your health and body. It happens slowly but surely. Therein lies the problem. People do not feel the impact of their poor choices until health problems occur much later on in the second half of life. By then, it can be too late.

High cholesterol levels, type 2 diabetes, blood pressure issues and countless other health problems are often a direct result of poor eating and a sedentary lifestyle.

One of the Most Fascinating Men in the World

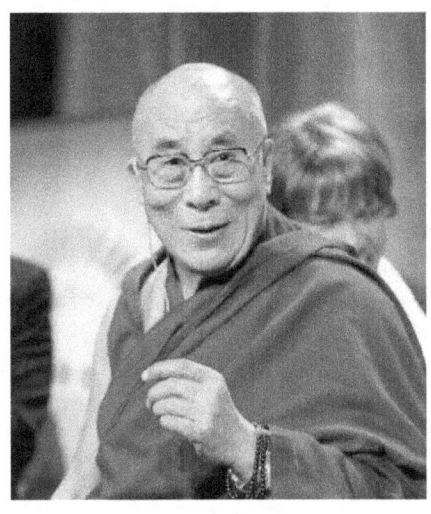

The Dalai Lama, when asked what surprised him most about humanity, answered, "Man.... Because he sacrifices his health in order to make money. Then he sacrifices money to recuperate his health. And then he is so anxious about the future that he does not enjoy the present; the result being that he does not live in the present or the future; he lives as if he is never going to die, and then dies having never really lived."

(*Photo credit – Christopher - Flickr: dalailama1_20121014_4639)

A wise man indeed. The point to note here is that while your career and family may be important, nothing supersedes your health.

From what you've read so far, it may seem to be all gloom and doom if you're guilty of having neglected your health for a while. Cast your fears aside. Your health and body constantly seek to improve and get better. You just need to assist them.

This finally brings us to the main point… Green smoothies. The miracle that even Popeye relied on. Technically, Popeye ate spinach. But you get the drift… Your greens are important for good health.

There is a movie titled, "Fat, Sick and Nearly Dead". You may have watched it, and if you've not, you might wish to check on YouTube to see if it has been uploaded there.

The movie is a real-life documentary about, Joe Cross, who was 100 lbs overweight and facing several serious health issues. Joe adopted a plant-based diet and mostly drank raw vegetable and fruit juices.

Within a few months, he had shed his excess weight and his health had improved by leaps and bounds. This certainly is testament to the power of a healthy diet.

There are several different types of smoothies which come in a range of different colors. In this guide, we'll be focusing on green smoothies which are without a doubt, the most powerful type of smoothies at restoring your health and vitality.

Are you sick and tired of feeling sick and tired? You are? Read on to find out how green smoothies will put you in the pink of health.

"When diet is wrong, medicine is of no use. When diet is correct, medicine is of no need." - **Ancient Ayurvedic Proverb**

Chapter 1 – Why greens?

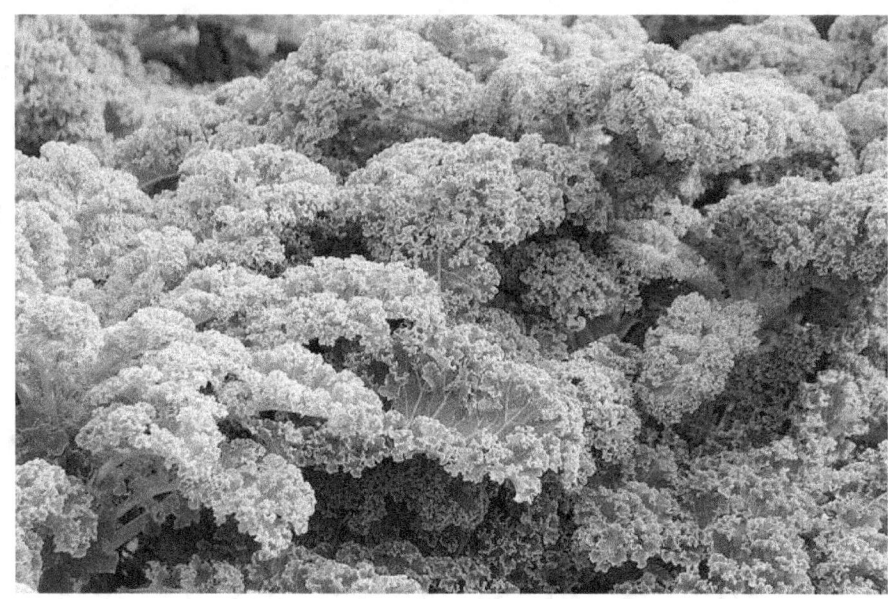

"Variety is the mother of enjoyment."

- Benjamin Disraeli

The first question that will pop into many people's minds when thinking of starting a juicing or smoothie diet will be, "Why are green smoothies better than other smoothies?"... After all, aren't all vegetables and fruits beneficial?

Yes, it's true that different fruit and vegetables contain a multitude of vitamins and antioxidants. However, greens contain a lot more vitamins and antioxidants than the other vegetables which are called "Phytonutrients". With a good mix of greens in your smoothies, you will not miss out on any vitamins that your body needs.

You should note that the drinks are made with raw vegetables and fruits. There are no additives, artificial flavouring, sugar or sweeteners, etc. The smoothies are best consumed in their raw form to derive the optimal benefits from the healthy, wholesome nutrients.

Now that we've discovered that green smoothies are a massive shortcut to excellent health & vitality, let's look at the benefits that can be accrued from preparing and consuming these smoothie gifts from nature.

Chapter 2 - Benefits of Green Smoothies

"It gets late early out there."

- Yogi Berra

Now we've discovered that green smoothies are excellent for one's health, let's look at how they actually help you get healthier and stronger.

- **Increased energy**

While you may not notice a change overnight, as you consume green smoothies over a period of 2 or 3 weeks, you'll notice that you have more energy and a better outlook in general. You will have more vitality and zest for life. You won't be able to explain why... but rest assured that the green smoothies are making a difference.

To achieve this, it's best to consume the smoothies on an empty stomach. Another good time to drink these smoothies is after an exercise session when your body is craving nutrients.

- **Aids in weight loss**

As mentioned earlier, Joe Cross lost almost 100 pounds from a juice fast. It may make many people panic when they think of not eating food and merely drinking smoothies. They fear starving or becoming under-nourished.

This is a huge fallacy. Our bodies require nutrients from food. That is true. However, there is a severe dearth of good nutrients in the food we consume these days. That is why people never feel satiated and constantly keep eating.

The food they're eating is high in processed ingredients, additives, etc. While it may fill the stomach, these are empty calories that lack the nutrients the body needs. As a result, the body craves more food to compensate for the lack of ingredients. So, people eat more, get obese and stay unhealthy.

Green smoothies are packed with micronutrients that the body craves. You would be surprised to learn that a single glass of green vegetable juice, full of good nutrients that the body craves, is more beneficial than an entire meal at a swanky restaurant.

- **They Combat and Prevent Illness**

This is pretty straightforward. Right from young, parents have instructed their children to eat their greens. Everyone knows that vegetables are essential for good health and for strengthening your immune system. Prevention is better than cure.

- **They Contain Healing Properties, Prevent Acne and Aid in Detoxification**

Green smoothies contain essential vitamins, minerals and nutrients that encourage quick healing. This is one reason why bodybuilders consume greens products. They usually take supplements in tablet form. Drinking green smoothies is much more beneficial than popping greens supplement tablets.

Acne sufferers, especially teenagers notice that their acne problems tend to diminish when consuming green juices. Since the greens are rich in vitamin A, sulphur, vitamin k, vitamin c, etc. the body's immune system is stronger and is able to combat health issues such as acne or even yeast infections effectively.

Detoxification is another fantastic benefit of green juices. The food we eat, water we drink and even the air we breathe is often filled with toxins. Green smoothies will help the body detoxify itself more effectively.

Other benefits:

- They are easily digested and the body is able to quickly assimilate the essential nutrients.

- The smoothies are rich in fiber and help maintain a healthy digestive system.

- They can be delicious once you get used to them. The mix of fruits and vegetables can be tasty. You're consuming a very tasty 'medicine' for your body.

- If you struggle to eat vegetables, green smoothies are a very convenient replacement. This applies to kids who hate eating vegetables. It is much easier to gulp down a green smoothie instead of gnawing on Brussels sprouts like a hamster at the dinner table.

They are just as healthy too. The smoothies, not the hamster.

- Green smoothies help to maintain a healthy cholesterol level in the body.

As you can see, you have nothing to lose and everything to gain by drinking green smoothies often.

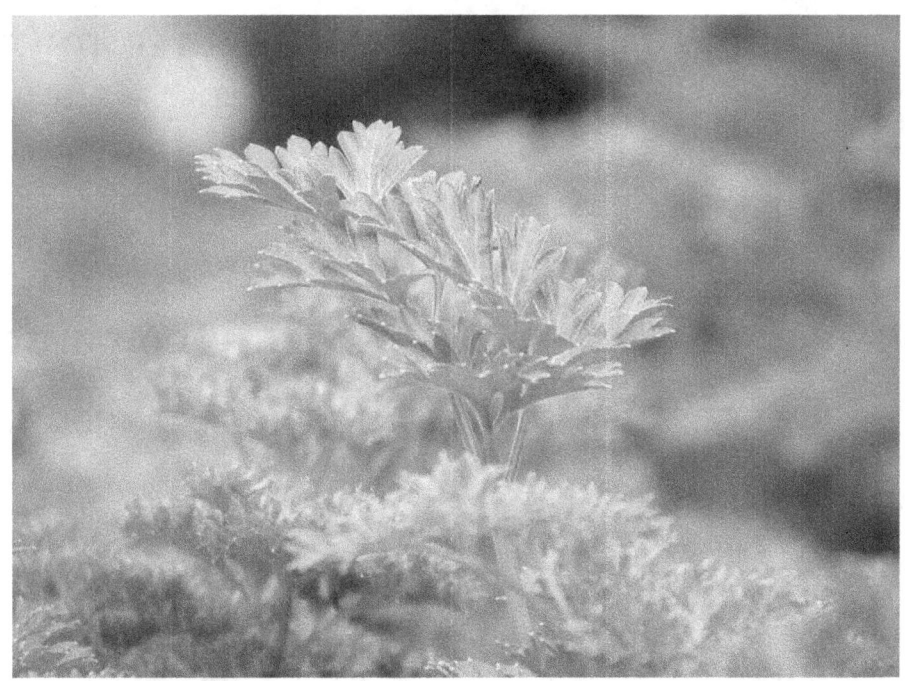

Chapter 3 – What are the Best Greens You Should Use

"Too many people are thinking of security instead of opportunity."

- James F. Byrnes

Not all green vegetables and fruits are created equal. When making a green smoothie, it's best to use vegetables that have the most nutrients to pack a punch. I mean, You want to get the best benefits from your smoothies.

Let's look at some of the best greens (in no particular order) that you can use to whip up those awesome smoothies.

- **Spinach**

Yup! Popeye was right. This truly is a fantastic green that is full of goodness. It is low in calories yet contains protein, iron, vitamins and minerals.

Spinach has been shown to lower the risk of cancer, strengthens bones, reduces the risk of asthma and other infections, lowers blood pressure and aids in glucose control for diabetics.

- **Kale**

Similar to spinach, kale is splendid for nourishing the body. In fact, kale contains more nutrients than spinach. It maintains healthy skin, strong bones, improves digestion and prevents the onset of many health problems.

- **Broccoli**

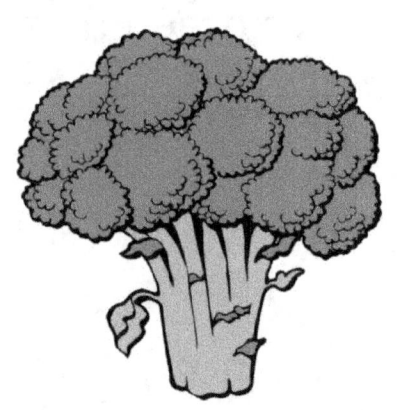

Broccoli is a cruciferous vegetable. It is fantastic for combating the effects of a poor diet. Our diets are rich in omega-6 fatty acids and this has thrown the balance of omega-3 and omega-6 fatty acids out of whack.

Our foods have become packed with estrogen, resulting in more men suffering from gynecomastia and other issues. Broccoli mitigates the negative effects of estrogen.

It's also rich in fiber and sulforaphane. This sulphur compound prevents cancers such as lung and colon cancer. Broccoli is definitely a vegetable that you should include in your smoothies often.

It does have a strong taste. So, start by using small amounts till you develop an acquired taste for it and are able to drink it without forcing yourself to.

- **Collards**

Collards are rich in vitamin K that promotes good bone health. They reduce the risks of developing colorectal, prostate and lung cancer. They also help diabetes sufferers maintain a stable blood glucose level.

An additional benefit of collard greens is that they contain choline. Choline helps with learning, memory, muscle movement and also promotes good sleep. Something which many people sorely need.

- **Cabbage**

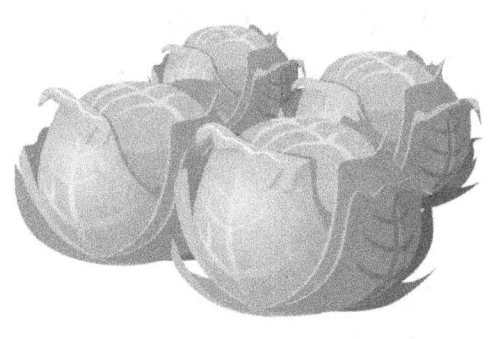

Cabbage is extremely low in calories but is high in fiber, protein, vitamin C and antioxidants. One cup of cabbage contains almost 50% of the average adult's daily vitamin C requirements.

It also contains manganese, potassium, calcium, folate, thiamine and vitamin B6. Antioxidants such as beta-carotene, lutein, etc. can also be found in cabbage.

You can reduce the risks of getting cancer, enhance your immunity, prevent cardiovascular disease and improve digestion by consuming cabbage.

- ## Celery

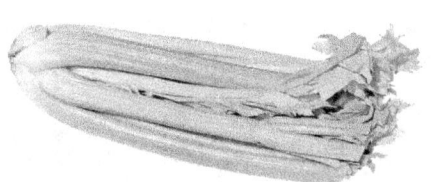

Just like the vegetables mentioned earlier, celery is rich in antioxidants, fiber, vitamins and minerals. It can prevent cancer and helps to lower one's blood pressure. One point to note is that some people are severely allergic to celery. Make sure you are not allergic to celery before consuming it.

- ## Dandelion Greens

Rich in vitamin C, iron, vitamin B6 and potassium. Also contains copper, folate, thiamine and phosphorous. Helps to good heart health and stabilise blood pressure levels.

- **Wheatgrass**

An excellent vegetable that is rich in many vitamins and nutrients. Prevents a whole host of health problems and also has healing properties.

- **Lettuce**

Fantastic for helping with weight loss. It is low in calories and reduces appetite. It contains many beneficial vitamins such as potassium, biotin, copper, calcium, panthothenic acid, chromium and magnesium.

Chapter 4 - Other beneficial greens you might want to look at.

"We don't want to get to the top of ladder to discover it was leaning against the wrong wall."

- Popular T-shirt Slogan

- **Parsley**

- **Chard**

- **Pak Choi/Bok Choy**

Are some greens better than others?

The most important point to remember is that eating any vegetable is better than eating none. The problem today is that most people are not even getting enough veggies in their diet... and French fries or mashed potatoes are NOT counted.

First and foremost, you need to get sufficient vegetables in your diet. If you do not like eating vegetables, you can make green smoothies. They are just as beneficial.

There is no need to worry if some greens are better than others because your goal will be to rotate the greens that you use in your smoothie. Some people make the exact same smoothie every single time and miss out on the benefits that they can get from the other vegetables.

Choose organic vegetables whenever you can. The hard truth is that most of our foods contain toxins from insecticides, fertilizers, etc. By rotating your greens, you will be preventing a toxin build-up from any one vegetable.

You should research what different green smoothie recipes there are. You can find many books in your library or at Amazon.com that contain many tasty and delicious green smoothie recipes.

These guides contain recipes created by nutritionists and health experts who have factored daily nutrient requirements, vegetable combinations, taste, etc. when concocting these recipes. You are in safe hands by following their recipes. The best way to stick with a habit is to like doing it.

Since the recipes will usually be tasty, you'll be more likely to stick to drinking smoothies instead of reaching for the sodas.

As long as you make smoothies from the vegetable list given above, or from a good recipe book, you will do just fine. This is not rocket science. It's just smoothies. Blend them and drink them. You will look and feel like a brand new you. It's that simple.

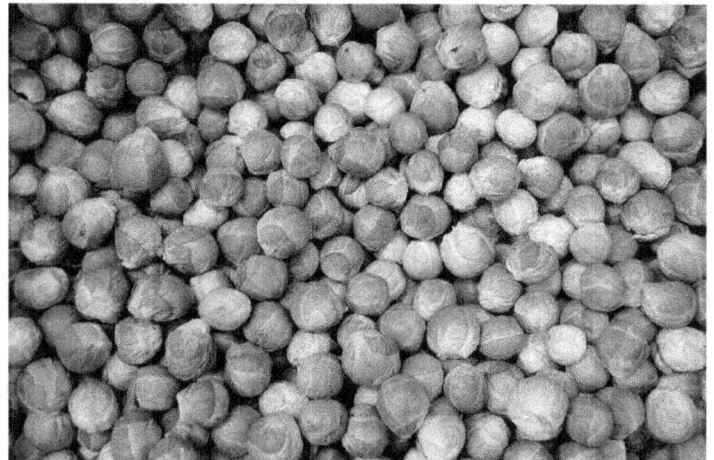

Chapter 5 – What are Smoothies and How Do You Make One

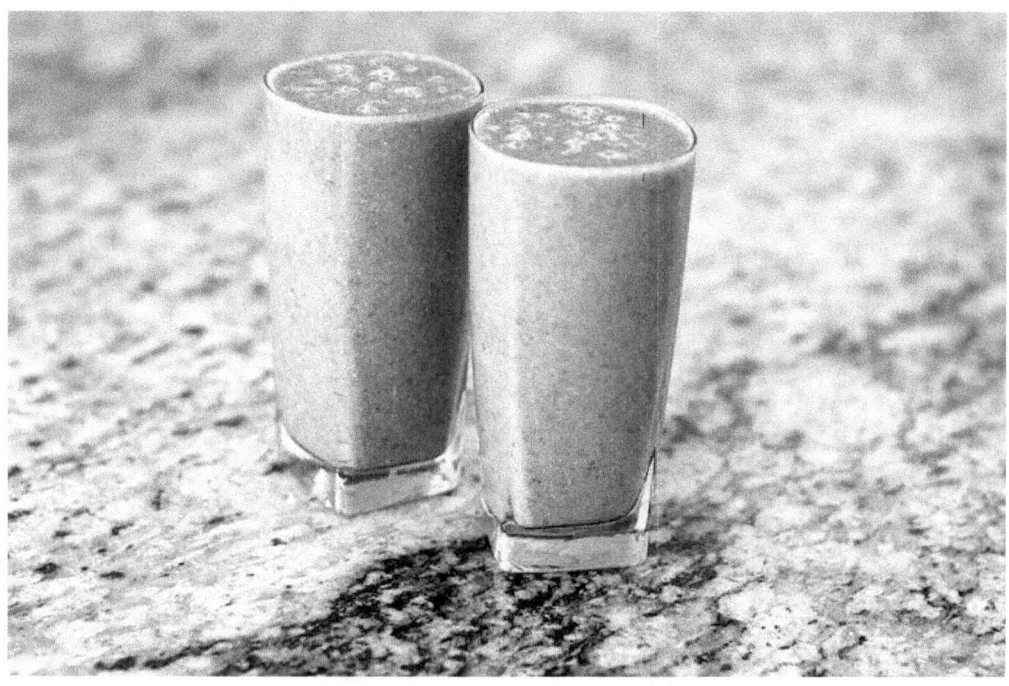

"Monotony is the awful reward of the careful."

- A.G. Buckham

It's funny we haven't yet covered it and we are half way through the guide! What exactly is a smoothie?

A smoothie is a thick beverage blend of different vegetables and fruits. Green smoothies use green vegetables such as spinach, celery cucumbers, green apples, etc.

The beauty of a smoothie is that you get many different nutrients, vitamins, minerals and antioxidants at one go. With the correct recipe, your smoothie will not only be healthy, but it will also be tasty. Many people believe that healthy food and tasty food cannot be reconciled. This is false. You can make a healthy and tasty smoothie.

Unlike normal smoothies, you will not be using yoghurt or milk to make your smoothie. The key here is to keep things natural. Many of the latest studies also show that milk and dairy products are not as beneficial as they were purported to be in the past. In fact, most are detrimental to one's health.

Since the goal here is to keep things raw and natural, the best way to make a smoothie will be to use chilled vegetables and fruit.

It has been shown that smoothies taste better when they are cold. It is better to use cold ingredients rather than to make a smoothie with vegetables at room temperature and chill it later on.

You will need good blender too. You can get one from your nearest appliance store or you could buy it online from Amazon (which goes without saying, do your research online first and make an informed decision as we all have different needs and budgets).

Add 2 or 3 cups of your green vegetables into the blender. Add 1 cup of water and if you have a sweet tooth, you can add some apple juice or pineapple juice to the mix. Turn on the blender/smoothie maker till you have a thick blend.

Congrats! You have a smoothie that's good to go.

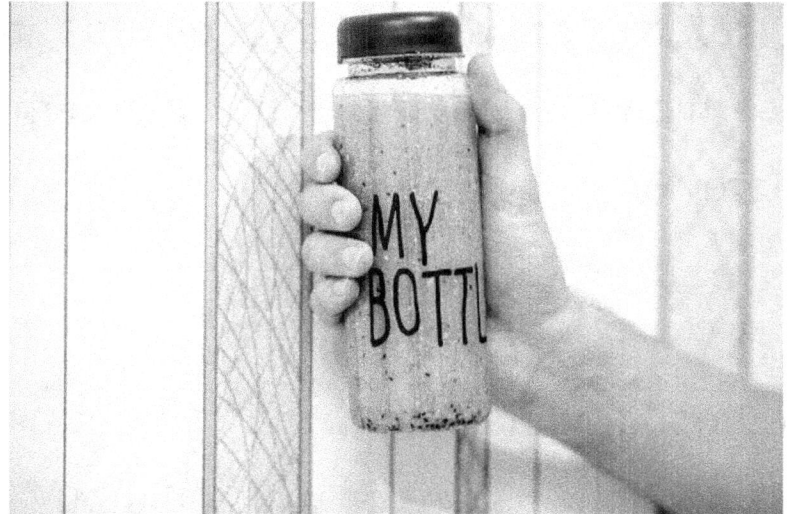

Chapter 6 – Are Smoothies Safe? What are the Common Mistakes to Avoid?

"We are always getting ready to live, but never living."

- Ralph Waldo Emerson

Smoothies are safe and beneficial to your health. However, they must be consumed in moderation. Anything that is taken to excess can be detrimental.

There are a few mistakes that people make unknowingly when making smoothies. The points below will shed light on the common mistakes and how to avoid them.

Mistake 1: Not rotating the greens

- Always rotate your greens. As mentioned in an earlier chapter, this will prevent toxin build-up and also give you a well-rounded smoothie diet.

Mistake 2: Not checking for allergies

- Be aware of your own allergies if you have any to vegetables and fruits. For example, some people are highly allergic to celery and can suffer from anaphylactic shock if they consume it. You might want to speak to your doctor about your green smoothie diet.

Mistake 3: Focusing on Fruits Instead of Veggies

- When making green smoothies, it is best to focus on the vegetables, rather than the fruits. It goes without saying that fruits are tastier because they are sweeter. Because of this, people usually use more fruits than green vegetables.

The problem here is that fruits are high in sugar but are not filling. You will not feel as satiated drinking a smoothie that is mostly fruit juice.

For example, if you make a green smoothie with:

- 1/2 cup of broccoli
- 1 banana
- ¾ cup blueberries
- ½ cup orange juice
- 1 cup strawberries
- 1 cup water

By all appearances, you have a green smoothie. Yes, this is good for your health but it will not leave you feeling full because it is low in fiber but high in natural sugars.

That basically means, you will get hungry sooner and end up eating more food to feel satiated. At the end of the day, you would have consumed more calories and will gain weight.

It is best to focus more on vegetables. Ideally, a good smoothie would look like this:

- ½ cup broccoli
- 1 cup spinach
- ½ cup cabbage
- 1 cup apple juice
- 1/2 cup water

Now you have a smoothie that is truly green, nutritious and the slow digesting fiber in the broccoli and spinach will leave you feeling full for longer.

Mistake 4: Not Keeping Things Natural

- Only use water and pure fruit juice when making your green smoothies. Using milk, yoghurt or store bought fruit juice is a big no-no.

There are several ingredients that people use thinking that these are nutritious and benefitting them. These are the most common ingredients added to green smoothies **which should be avoided**.

1. Protein powder
2. Ice cream
3. Sugar
4. Cream soda
5. Honey
6. Whipped cream
7. Peanut butter
8. Chocolate syrups

There is one cardinal rule to making smoothies. No artificial ingredients. You should only use green vegetables and a few small servings of raw fruit or natural fruit juice to make the smoothie. The fruits just help to make the drink sweeter and more palatable. No deviation from this rule. Period.

Mistake 5: Not Using a Good Blender

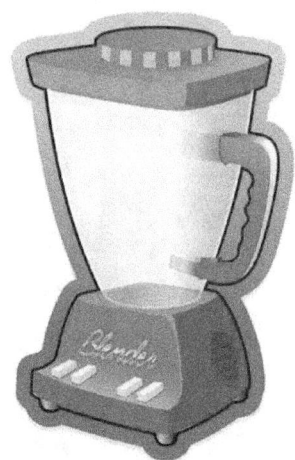
While this is not a huge mistake, it is still better to use good blender rather than one ill-suited for making smoothies.

The blender should have a solid base that is wide for stability. Since you're making smoothies with your blender, it needs to have a high-speed and a 1000+ watt motor.

The pitcher that the blender uses needs to be large too. Sometimes you may want to make a smoothie for 2 or more people. At times like these, you will need a bigger blender rather than a small, personal one.

Do your research and see what is the best type of juicer for you and is within your budget.

Mistake 6: Not Using Proper Recipes

 Do not try to concoct your own recipes. There are thousands of recipes available online or in books for you to copy. Using too many veggies in your blend will make it have a muddy appearance and the flavors may not be complementary.

Many beginners do not know that certain greens such as arugula and broccoli have a strong taste. You'll need to know what ingredients can mask the taste of these vegetables. It's best to stick to recipes written by the pros.

Chapter 7 - 7 Healthy and Yummy Smoothie

Recipes for Seniors

"Everything that is done in the world is done by HOPE."

- Martin Luther

The best time to drink a smoothie will be upon waking. The second best time to drink a smoothie will be after a workout session. Do make regular exercise a part of your lifestyle and finish it off with a tall, cold glass of green juice?

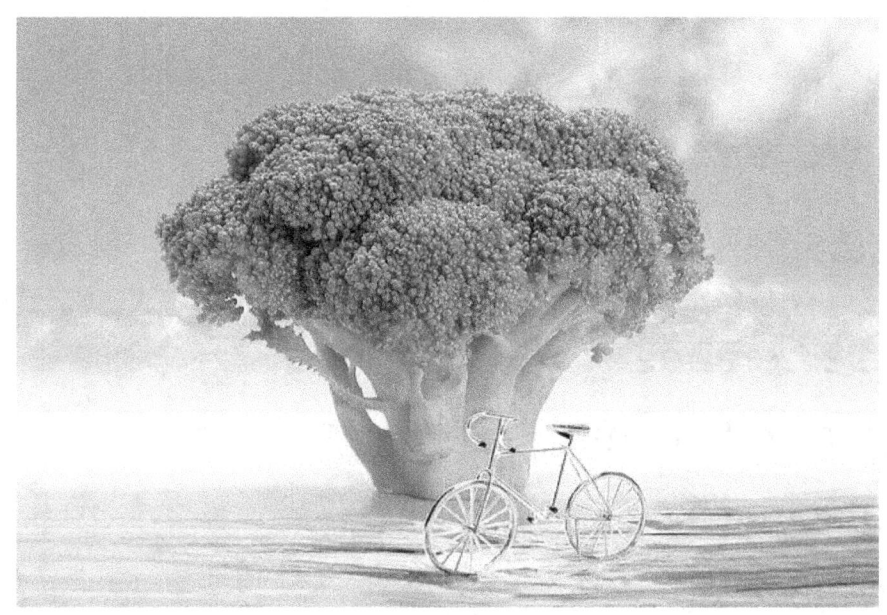

If you can't drink your smoothies during these times, then any other time will do just fine. What really matters is that you are making and drinking the green smoothies. Implementation is half the battle won. You do not have to be perfect when you start. Just start and then aim to improve as you progress.

Below, you will find 7 green smoothie recipes. All recipes serve 1 person. You can drink them at any time of the day. These are tasty, nutritious recipes. Make sure you're not allergic to any of the ingredients before making them.

Recipe 1: Orange Spinach Surprise

Ingredients:

- 1 peeled orange
- 1/2 peeled banana
- 1 cup spinach
- 1/2 cup water
- 1 tsp flaxseed

- Ice cubes

Directions:

Add all the ingredients into the blender and ice cubes as required. Blend till you get the desired consistency. Pour into a glass and drink away.

Recipe 2: Green Avocado Smoothie

Ingredients:

- 1/2 cup pineapple chunks
- 1/2 avocado, diced
- 1 cup (2 handfuls) fresh spinach
- 1/2 cup coconut water
- 1 tablespoon hemp seeds
- 1 frozen, sliced banana

Directions:

Blend all the ingredients to desired consistency and serve chilled

Recipe 3: Green Detox Smoothie

Ingredients:

- 1 cup organic kale
- 1/2 cup parsley
- 1 cup cucumber
- 1/2 cup pineapple
- 1 lemon
- 1/2 avocado
- 1 cup unsweetened green tea
- 1 tablespoon fresh grated ginger

Directions:

Squeeze the juice from the lemon into the blender.

Add the rest of the ingredients and blend to desired consistency

Recipe 4: Romaine Lettuce Smoothie

Ingredients

- 1 cup water
- 1 chopped apple
- 1 cup organic, chopped romaine lettuce
- 1/2 cup spinach
- 1/2 cup chopped celery
- 1/2 frozen, sliced banana
- 1 chopped pear

Directions:

Add lettuce, spinach and water and blend till you get a smooth mix. Add rest of the ingredients except the banana into blender.

Blend till required consistency. Add in banana and blend till the beverage is smooth. Pour and drink.

Recipe 5: Kale Kissed by Ginger Smoothie

Ingredients:

- 2 large kale leaves
- 1/2 bunch of parsley

- 1/2 cup cucumber
- 1/2 cup pineapple chunks
- 1/2 apple
- 1 cup celery
- 1/2 cup water
- 1 tablespoons grated ginger

Directions:

Place all ingredients into blender and blend till desired consistency.

Recipe 6: Kool Kiwi Spinach Smoothie

Ingredients:

- 1 cup spinach
- 1 cup strawberries
- 1 cup cucumber
- 1 tsp hemp seeds (optional)
- 1 sliced, frozen banana
- 1 cup kiwi fruit

- 1 cup water

Directions:

Add all ingredients into blender and blend to desired consistency. Best served chilled.

Recipe 7: Tropical Smoothie Dream

Ingredients:

- 1/2 cup parsley
- 1/2 cup cucumber
- 1/2 banana sliced & frozen
- 1 stalks celery
- 1 cup pineapple chunks
- 1/2 cup peaches
- 1/2 tsp grated ginger
- 1 cup coconut water cucumber

Directions:

Blend all the ingredients in blender till desired consistency is achieved, and serve chilled.

Green Smoothies for Seniors

Conclusion – How to Make Smoothies a Part of Your Life

"We first make our habits. Then our habits make us."

– John Dryden

Wow, we've reached the conclusion of our introductory guide to Green Smoothies and you're still here...Great achievement.

But as we know, information is only the first step...next is implementation so If you're not in the habit of drinking smoothies, you will need to cultivate the habit first. You can start with 1 smoothie a day. Do not worry about the time you consume it.

If you can consume it first thing in the morning, that would be great. If you can't, later on in the day will do fine. What's important is that you get into the habit of drinking one a day.

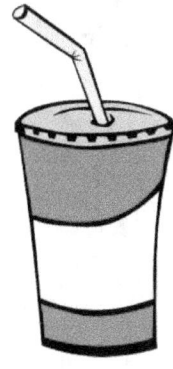 Let's face the facts here. Despite what the books and nutritionists say, most smoothies though tasty will never come close to a sugary soda or an ice cream milk shake. That's the hard truth. It will be difficult to replace sodas with smoothies.

Initially, you may wish to slowly cut down on any sugary drinks you're consuming and drink a smoothie every day. Over time, try and replace the sodas with the smoothies. It will take effort but if you approach it in a slow and steady manner, it can be done.

Do not go to extremes and immediately give up all the sodas for smoothies. You'll just be putting pressure and stress on yourself. Now, not only are you trying to inculcate a good habit that is foreign to you but you've also given up a bad habit that brought you comfort despite being detrimental to your health.

This is just too much to cope with. You're not in a race. Go slow and your compliance will be much higher. Inch by inch, life's a cinch. Yard by yard, life is hard.

If you're trying to lose weight, you can try to replace one of your meals with a smoothie. The smoothie may not be as satisfying as a normal meal such as a plate of pasta or 3 slices of pizza, but it will be much better for your health.

Aim to do this just once a day till you're comfortable with it. Then you may progress to reducing your meal portion sizes and even replacing 2 meals with smoothies. If you can do this, your fat will melt like butter and you will drop the pounds in no time at all.

If you're a parent, you can start your child on smoothies while they are young. Most children do not like eating vegetable but will hastily gulp down a tall smoothie if it had apple juice in it. They will still be getting all the vegetable nutrients without you having to negotiate and debate with them at the dinner table.

While green smoothies are excellent for your health, occasionally you may wish to try other smoothies too. The rules are not set in stone and you're not in a green smoothie prison. Though this book did focus solely on green smoothies, you can always give the rest a try, as long as you're drinking 1 green smoothie daily.

Usually, it is recommended that green smoothies should be comprised of 60% fruits and 40% veggies. This is a good place to start with but over time, you should progress to 60% or 70% vegetables and 40% or 30% fruits respectively.

The reason for this is that most people these days are carrying more fat on their bodies than they should. By increasing the vegetable intake and reducing the fruits, you'll be consuming less sugar. Your body will burn more fat and you'll lose any excess weight even faster.

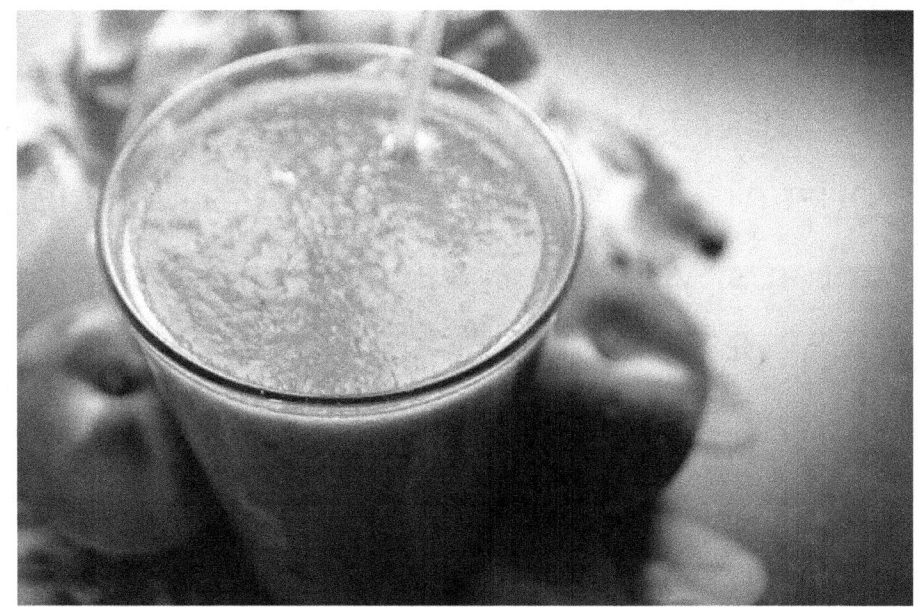

The benefits of green smoothies are many. By now, you should be fully aware that you'd be doing yourself a disservice by not drinking them. Like Hippocrates said, "Let food be thy medicine and medicine be thy food." Green smoothies are your medicine.

It may take a while to develop the habit... but persist anyway. The green smoothie lifestyle is definitely something you want to have. The rewards are fantastic!

SNEAK PREVIEW of:

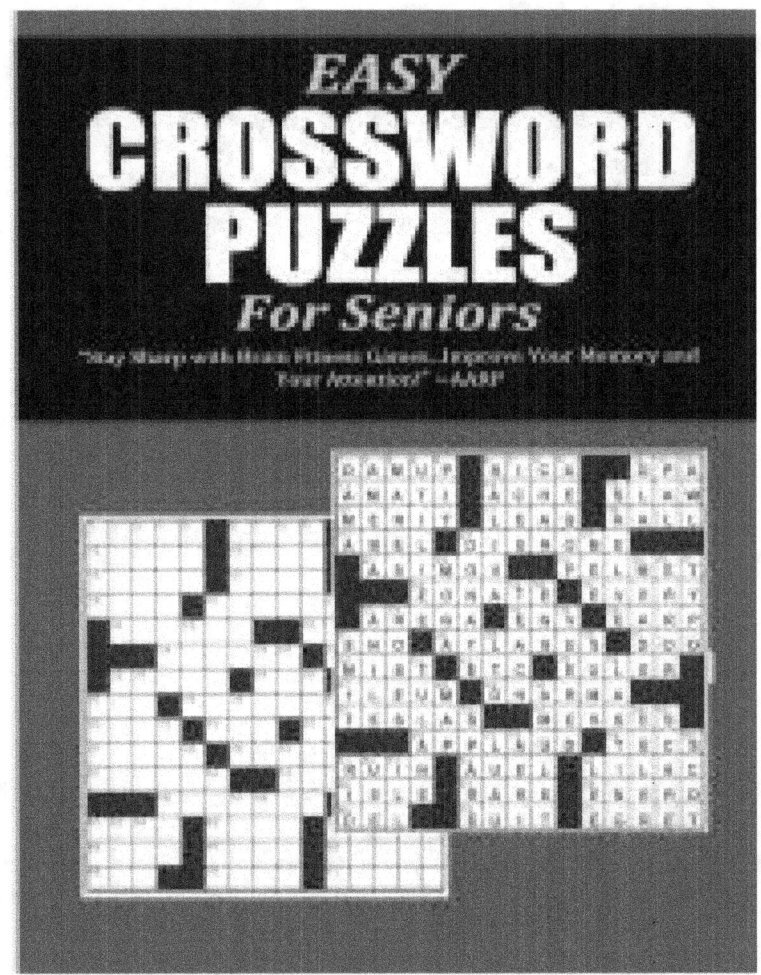

Order your copy online today at:

EASY CROSSWORD

PUZZLES

For

Seniors

ACROSS

1- Advised
9- Lets up
15- Substance for killing rats
16- Shipworm
17- Ambiguous
18- Dried grape
19- Used to be
20- Small piece of lean meat
22- 1957 hit for the Bobbettes
26- Curved sword
27- Trident-shaped letter
29- Actor Byrnes
30- Latin 101 word
31- Betrothed
33- Deadly
38- Willingly
39- Divided, anatomically
41- Japanese form of fencing
42- Muslim opponent of the Crusaders
43- Writer Hentoff
46- Uno + due
47- Worked (up)
48- Purplish red
52- With cunning
54- Imitates
56- Joie de vivre
59- Charlotte ___, Virgin Islands
60- Prototype
64- Inn
65- Excited
66- Caught
67- Cocks

DOWN

1- Get one's ducks in ___
2- Trim
3- Grouse
4- Kitchen gadget
5- Hosp. section
6- Part of RSVP
7- Writer LeShan
8- "Jurassic Park" actress
9- Skylighted lobby
10- Predatory mammal
11- Disney mermaid
12- Seed covering
13- Prepares for publication
14- Loudness units
21- South American tuber
23- Member of a French foreign corps
24- Pulitzer-winning biographer Leon
25- Whirlpool
27- Enliven
28- Dagger of yore
32- Find the sum of
34- Loss leader?
35- Form of basalt
36- Fit to ___
37- Pre-Easter season
39- Fast fliers
40- British nobleman
44- Be present
45- ___ kwon do
48- Deli offerings
49- Capital of Jordan
50- Tropical fruit
51- "Oklahoma!" aunt
53- Sic on
55- River to the Moselle
57- Impersonator
58- Actor Beatty and others
61- Vietnam's ___ Dinh Diem
62- Juan's uncle
63- UFO pilots

Crossword puzzle grid (answers filled in):

1 A	2 P	3 P	4 R	5 I	6 S	7 E	8 D	■	9 A	10 B	11 A	12 T	13 E	14 S
15 R	A	T	I	C	I	D	E	■	16 T	E	R	E	D	O
17 O	R	A	C	U	L	A	R	■	18 R	A	I	S	I	N
19 W	E	R	E	■	■	20 N	21 O	I	S	E	T	T	E	
■	■	22 M	R	23 L	24 E	25 E	26 C	U	T	L	A	S	S	
27 P	28 S	I	■	29 E	D	D	30 A	M	O	■				
31 E	N	G	32 A	G	E	D	■		33 F	34 A	35 T	36 A	37 L	
38 R	E	A	D	I	L	Y	■	39 S	40 E	P	T	A	T	E
41 K	E	N	D	O	■		42 S	A	R	A	C	E	N	
■			43 N	44 A	45 T	46 T	R	E	■	47 H	E	T		
48 M	49 A	50 G	51 E	N	T	A	52 S	L	Y	53 L	Y	■		
54 E	M	U	L	A	T	E	55 S	■		56 E	L	57 A	58 N	
59 A	M	A	L	I	E	■	60 A	61 N	62 T	63 E	T	Y	P	E
64 T	A	V	E	R	N	■	65 A	G	I	T	A	T	E	D
66 S	N	A	R	E	D	■	67 R	O	O	S	T	E	R	S

www.ingramcontent.com/pod-product-compliance
Lightning Source LLC
Chambersburg PA
CBHW080833310526
45788CB00020B/3517